Other poetry books written by the author are as follows:

Love, Hate, Infatuation, Betrayal
Life, Memories, and Dreams
The Colours of Life, Seasonal Gifts

ON BEING SCHIZOAFFECTIVE— A SURREAL SOUL

Understand the Experience of Being Low,
High, Anxious, and Psychotic—
An Existential View

AMANDA JAYNE GILMER

authorHOUSE®

AuthorHouse™ UK
1663 Liberty Drive
Bloomington, IN 47403 USA
www.authorhouse.co.uk
Phone: UK TFN: 0800 0148641 (Toll Free inside the UK)
*   UK Local: 02036 956322 (+44 20 3695 6322 from outside the UK)*

Published by AuthorHouse 01/30/2021

ISBN: 978-1-6655-8523-1 (sc)
ISBN: 978-1-6655-8524-8 (e)

Print information available on the last page.

CONTENTS

Introduction vii

Mental Illness, Existentialism, and Me 1
Surreal Soul 3
Writing the Blues 4
Pitter-Patter 5
Poetry 6
Without a Cause 7
Tired 8
A Prayer for Me 9
Spirit Walker 10
Pass Me By 11
Out of the Dark and Into the Light 12
Not Afraid 13
Joy 14
Empty 15
Demons and Shadows 16
Cry 17
The Night 18
The Loft 19
The Reaper's Call 20
New Moon Rising 21
Demons 22
Runaway Life 23
Alive 24
Black Shadows 25

Mental Illness 26
A Bond 27
The Dagger and The Serpent 29
When I Lost My Mind 30

Author's Note 33

INTRODUCTION

The author was diagnosed with schizoaffective disorder eight years ago after suffering a breakdown. This pamphlet explores the illness and how it affected her. She is hoping other sufferers of severe mental illness will relate to the poems within, which explore depression, anxiety, and being high and low.

Schizoaffective disorder pairs the highs and lows of bipolar disorder with the psychosis of schizophrenia. Many aspects of the author's illness were unexplainable and difficult to understand. Poetry enabled her to explain and explore these elements in the written word. Her illness was previously not spoken about, and these poems helped her come to terms with her experiences.

She also wants to convey that there is life after mental breakdown and that recovery is possible. For her, poetry was a part of this.

MENTAL ILLNESS, EXISTENTIALISM, AND ME

The Courage to Be, by existential philosopher Paul Tillich, explains how we need to be true to ourselves and accept ourselves without shame or reproach. Stereotypes and prejudice can be blocks to this and lead to shame—particularly when it comes to mental illness.

You should not be overly concerned by others' perceptions. Only you truly know yourself. Much of human behaviour is directed at closing the existential gap we perceive and feel. One must strive to understand one's own being in the world and that of others.

Angst and anxiety are part of life, as is the realisation that we are free to choose our own paths. But the ways in which we choose our paths are up to us. Mental illness complicates this. It can often heighten anxiety. It can also lead to denial, false perceptions, blame, and hate as we cannot accept this responsibility.

When a person has a mental illness, the existential gap is far wider than it is for those without mental illness. The experience of mental illness is far more removed from everyday experience. This can lead to stigma based on hate, prejudice, and stereotypes. Understanding and closing the existential gap on an individual and a societal level is important in enabling people to deal with the devastating impact of mental illness.

I have been diagnosed with schizoaffective disorder, a severe mental illness that has as its symptoms both the psychosis of schizophrenia and the highs and lows of bipolar disorder. This book was written for my mum, Dorothy Louisa Gilmer, who has stood by my side through thick and thin, always there whether she understood or not. She wanted to understand, and this is my book to her.

The book has its roots in phenomenology and is my meaning, from my subjective point of view. It aims to close the existential gap and explores the experience of being high, low, anxious, and psychotic.

This book is intended to develop understanding and insight for family, friends, coworkers, professionals, or anyone who has an interest in mental health. It was also written for others who have experienced mental health complications, to enhance their understanding and being in this often-challenging world.

SURREAL SOUL

A surreal soul hiding in the dark, cast amongst the shadows, contemplating her plight. A mind full of magic, a heart full of woe. The shadows are closing as her heart screams out. Why does it have to be this way? The world is unwelcoming as she lives in her daydream whilst still awake. Feeling all alone—a scary place that shakes her soul.

A broken mind, ethereal dreams whilst still awake. Weary but still strong. The nightmare world is now a chapter to be closed. But with a lasting memory ... why did it go so wrong? A lonely world no one could understand.

Paliperidone, the bringer of light, freed my soul from the monsters plaguing me and eating at my soul—lightened my heart and my mind. I came in from the dark. I am no longer broken, freed from the demons that haunted my shattered mind.

WRITING THE BLUES

The blues is your ruler. A rollercoaster ride that only goes down. Nothing can stop it or make a difference. The ride does not let up till it has decided to halt. Depression will be your foe till its time is done.

It will take your self-respect and your sense of pride. The birds are singing, but you are sinking, a belly full of dread. The morning time is ticking, but you cannot stop thinking. Oh, just go back to bed. The afternoon's here; nothing's done. Cannot seem to focus or push yourself on. Cannot shake that feeling that's with you all day long.

There is no let-up; there is no cause. A prison of black—there is no escaping. It colours your thoughts, emotions, and feelings. I write in vain as I feel the same. Writing the blues—a chronicle to the darkness of my pain.

The thing that keeps you going is that you know it will pass. Another day is looming, hoping this is the day it will pass—when the black dog retreats and the blues pass once again.

PITTER-PATTER

I can hear the raindrops as I contemplate. Another night not sleeping; I feel so awake. I love this eerie hour; for me it's time to get things done. I put my thoughts into rhyme as the rain gently drops, *pitter-patter*—the soundtrack to my words.

Still, the night. I love the quiet and peacefulness as I begin to write. The thoughts are flowing; I had better write this down.

The raindrops relax me and are soothing to my mind. Writing at this untimely hour is a feature of my life. My mind is sharp and focused as I write away. Still, the night.

Another night. My creativity has found its urge to the beat of *pitter-patter* as the raindrops fall. Still, the night, as I contemplate.

POETRY

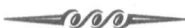

Poetry is my love; poetry became my life. With the little ups and downs, it makes a nine-to-five hard to keep down. Writing became my solace; it kept boredom from my door. I expressed my life in many ways and loved exploring it in rhyme.

It gave expression to many endless thoughts. Eventually it gained purpose, and I put my words into books. I now have a sense of pride and achievement I never thought I could attain. Each book is different and reflects different aspects of my life. Poetry enabled me to bring my thoughts to life, exploring things I never talked about.

I still have my troubles, but I have something I can do. The enjoyment I have in the written word could never be replaced. It gives me a sense of purpose as well as self-belief.

Poetry is my love and my life—an expression that will last forever, and a legacy for my sons.

WITHOUT A CAUSE

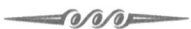

It does not need a cause or reason; it just occurs—a withering of the soul. Without a will, without a soul.

Once my eyes shone so bright. But now my heart is blighted; everything's slow.

Weary-hearted.
Mind cannot think.
My heart is heavy.

I cannot think straight; just keep wondering about those pearly gates. Senseless, hopeless, and without reason. But why? Messed-up brain needs some serotonin to take away the pain.

The black dog comes and goes—a testimony to the pointless. God, I feel like a waste of space. No joy, no lift: a place I cannot escape. The blues come out of the blue—out of nowhere—the darkest bolt piercing my ravaged soul.

Everything is pressure; there is no getting it together. Close the bedroom door; close my eyes. Soon it will be light.

TIRED

Scared of dying. Tired of life. Everything is full of dread. Avoiding people, solace my only goal.

My anxiety is overbearing—a tightness in my chest. I cannot stop thinking. Worrying about nothing at all. Negative thoughts fill my mind.

My heart is heavy.
My mind racing.
My soul unsettled.

Nervous and on edge. Wringing hands. Hollow eyes. So restless at night. Counting sheep. Another hour passes by. Insomnia's here … God, how I dread the night. Daybreak's here. So tired, but the thoughts will not leave my mind.

Anxiety passes. I will love the night again. I am waiting for the time when I have a truly settled mind.

My belly is no more full of dread. The fog has lifted, my thoughts no longer bleak. When I shut my eyes, I gently nod and wake up refreshed to face the day. The tightness in my chest has gone away.

A PRAYER FOR ME

O Lord, my saviour, deliver me from this wretched life that no one can understand. Please close the rifts inside my mind so I can see joy and light again. Please heal my tortured soul and calm the storm beneath. The disturbance in my mind needs protection from above. I hold my cross every day, waiting for the day I will be healed and be the person I was.

Protect me from the demons that haunt my mind and that I see so vividly. Take away the voices that relentlessly talk to me. This is a prayer for myself to take away the haunting in my life and the monsters that I see. They seem so true to life, but all I want is my normal life back. So answer my prayer soon. I still believe in you, despite the torture in my soul and the pain that blackens my heart.

A prayer to heal. A prayer to feel. Take me back to that happy place where my mind was free of the demons consuming me. I will wait for the day my mind is truly free and no longer lost in the ethereal world to be truly at peace.

SPIRIT WALKER

You are the spirits that walk the earth. My soul came to life. A shadowy outline. Voices closing in after dark. Day walkers, night walkers. The spirit world consumed my mind—an eerie world that came to life in my home and as I walked.

My life is passing me by, but I am at one with the afterlife. Visions so real—a scary world. The spirit world has come to life.

I can see their shadows; I can hear their voices. Is this spiritual enlightenment or a fragmented mind unravelling before my eyes? Is this dark world a figment of my shattered mind, or another dimension that came to life, the end result of a shattered soul?

The shadows encroach, but my mind needs peace. When will this enlightenment of the spirit end? Another weary night. It is morning now and time to sleep. The demon world has stolen my night once again.

PASS ME BY

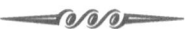

Watching the world pass me by, I feel so numb I cannot even cry. I watch them get on with their day to day. I want to feel the same. For me it is a chore even getting out of bed these days. But I just reframe and wait for it to end. Waiting for the day, I feel shiny again.

It passes, as it always does. So just hold on; the feeling will end. There will be a time when I feel joyous again. I have watched the world pass me by, but now I am ready to be with it again.

The tunnel is long and can consume, but happiness can be yours again. Remember: the feeling goes. Just keep going; there is light at the end. I will beat it once again.

OUT OF THE DARK AND INTO THE LIGHT

I lost the light, and the shadows encroached. To see the light, to feel the high, I need to take the night. Oh, what it is to feel this bright dancing in the light—a feeling that got lost amongst the shadows. It has put an end to my dreary plight.

Happy and warm, ready to face the world. A rosy feeling, full of warmth, offsets the chilly feeling of being in the dark.

Creativity at a peak. Full of ideas. Need to write them down. A gentle up—welcome relief. Now I am getting up to speed. This lovely feeling always ends. But I remember the joy to see me through life's cruel twist again. Out of the dark and into the light; now I feel the night, no longer scared of the dark.

NOT AFRAID

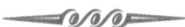

Let the haters hate. Where is the shame? I embrace what I am. The struggle within my mind made me what I am.

Watch me rise; I will touch the sky. There is no stopping now; I am rolling like I am high. I am not afraid to be what I am. Truth-teller or liar? In the end, no one's gonna give a damn.

Creativity. A razor-sharp mind. An empathy for others you cannot replicate. Energy as awesome as a hurricane. A disease of the mind that illuminates and expands the normal limitations that tend to encase a person's mind.

Mayhem is my middle name. Mischief and fun is the name of the game. Do not be afraid; vulnerability is only a weakness to those that hate. It is a gift that sets your heart free.

Let the world join hands and embrace life with affection and warmth. Compassion is the key; and love, the enemy of hate.

Defender of the light fighting back from the dark, let the millions unite who fought to leave a dark place. Life can be surprising, even though it sometimes hurts. No one ever has to be afraid

JOY

Happiness in my heart, joy in my soul, softness in my mind. Life just feels so good. The singing of birds, the humming of bees. I'm noticing everything in nature's garden; the lambs frolic and play.

Little things seem to bring such joy. The trees are swaying in the breeze; the sky is so blue. I am waiting upon dusk to see the stars peeping through. Such a beautiful starlit night. The moon luminescent and full, so still the night. What a feeling as I look above. I hold on to this feeling to help me through the dark that can sometimes consume my heart.

EMPTY

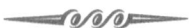

I gazed at the world from an empty place, wondering, "How?" Wondering "When? When will there be an end?" A sorrowful existence. Watching the world pass me by. Nothing is right; everything is wrong. This deceptive feeling from deep within.

A black shadow—no longer the person I was. How do I stop this black facade? When will I feel joy? This is a feeling I cannot explain that is so alien to me.

Black like a raincloud, unsettled and bleak. Waiting for the sunshine to peep through and the rain to end. Every so often, there is a little ray—a sign that joy will be in my heart again.

It ends, as it always does, and sunshine pours into that empty place. A sunny heart will be mine again, and life will be just as it should.

I smile, but no longer with tears behind my eyes, as the blackness turns to joy.

DEMONS AND SHADOWS

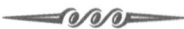

The night is still. I can hear the whispers. I feel cold and clammy. The mist is drawing in. The voices are getting closer. Their silhouettes are shadowy as their shadows move, glistening in the moonlight. My mind is full of dread at their voices being inside my head.

Praying for the morning, I clutch my chest. I can hear my heartbeat on this eerie night. Voices are all around me as their shadows move. The darkness is upon me; I can feel the fear.

The morning is approaching; the shadows are retreating. No more Voices inside my head. The dawn is breaking; now I can get some rest. The fearful night has ended. I no longer have the tightness in my chest.

The day has quickly ended; dusk is fast approaching. Shadows fall across my window, my belly full of dread. I can hear their voices—the demons inside my head. The night-time is steadily more fearful with each passing day.

The cross is my defender and protector from the night creatures trying to steal my soul.

CRY

I cried a river; my soul shone blue. It is happening again, like a bolt from the blue. No hazard warning. I feel so confused. The breath of darkness is withering my soul.

Just last week, I felt true joy. This up-and-down roller coaster is all it seems to be. Just try to remember there will be a breaking dawn. The low will disappear as quickly as it came. But it feels like forever—like it will never end.

A blanket of black, a glass full of sorrow. How do I feel so empty? I cannot face the morning, lingering in bed. It is a feeling so consuming that I cannot escape. I am so full of dread, so I just give up instead, waiting for it to end and for the rain from heaven to clear my damaged mind.

I tell myself it is a cycle and it will end in time. Crying silently on my own, I feel so ashamed. I pull the duvet over and try to relax my mind. It will soon be over; I will smile again. The thorny crown of self-loathing will disappear once again.

THE NIGHT

This is the night. This is the light. This is the right. But is this the wrong that will be the right?

Just one dance.
Just one trance.
Just one look.

No need to explain. Only feel, only trust; do not blink. A synergy of energy. My perfect quest.
Wrong time, wrong mind.
Right time, right mind.

Fuzzy mind, head closed up. Need to be opened, need to be free. Eyes lit like the sunlight on the brightest day. Shine like the moonlight sky, waiting for shooting stars to collide.

THE LOFT

Smoky and dark but loud and bright. A place to lose your mind. A place to shake your soul. All night bump and grind, the liquor flowing strong. What a buzz, dancing all night long.

The music is great; I cannot wait to shake all night long. The people come and go, putting on their private shows.

A place to lose your mind; a place to shake your soul. The loft is such a high; the enjoyment lasts all night long. There's something different every week—oh, what a show. I want to levitate to the DJ's set; everyone is shiny-eyed.

What a place to go—a smoky den filled with all walks of life. A pleasure till the end. Now it is 4 a.m., time to go. Stress relieved, dancing till the end.

THE REAPER'S CALL

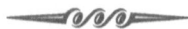

I can hear the reaper; he is knocking at my door. Shadows fall outside my window. Can you hear his call? Dark shadows are everywhere, so I no longer go out at night. I see things after dark.

So scared the reaper will call, I am drawing perfect circles everywhere to protect myself from harm, clutching the cross to protect me from what's a figment of my mind.

I can hear the reaper; he is knocking at my door. Shadows outside my window, shadows when I walk. I used to feel free and love the night. Now it is full of shadows—the twilight world I dread.

I am waiting for the break of dawn so I can go to bed. The night shift is over; now it is time for sleep—till the next night, when I fear the reaper will call and slip inside my home.

This is an imaginary world only I can see, but the fear is real. I prayed to God to save my soul as the night just left me froze.

My mind let in the ethereal world, but now I have saved my soul. The twilight world has left me; I can sleep alone. It was a world only my eyes could see. My special power: seeing a world full of make-believe.

NEW MOON RISING

There is a new moon rising. I am shining—never felt so good. My heart is soaring; good times are here to stay. After the blues of yesterday and all the reeling, I am finally healing.

There is a new moon rising. My eyes are gleaming, full of sparkly fun. I thought I would never recover from the madness of it all. Like the full moon, I have never shone so bright.

Now I am living life to the full. No more dreading, just chilling and loving the day. Anxiety, paranoia, hallucinations, and high-to-low was the order of the day. Two years have passed, and I am still settled, looking forward to the start of each new day.

The new moon is rising. I have fallen in love with the night once again. The nightmare has ended; my reality is back to normal once again.

DEMONS

I have no need to roar; there is no cause. The demons have left my home again. The stress has gone away. I am feeling more robust, my life truly settled; there are only minor hiccups with gentle ups and downs.

I have no need to roar; there is no cause. Life was once a roller coaster ride, and my monsters came to life—a paranormal vision, a nightmare whilst awake.

I had lots of imaginary friends, and the monsters too. I heard their voices all the time and saw them in my visions too. The inanimate came to life; I could speak to objects too. My ornaments talked to me—my imaginary kingdom in my magical, mythical world.

Demons in my dreams, demons in the night—they came to me in voices and hallucinations too. Demons in the windowpanes tried to get inside my house. My home is full of precious things to stop the demons getting in and overtaking my world.

Now that my psychosis has come to pass, I have no need to roar. I just pause and take a breath. A chapter of my life has closed shut. I am no longer dreaming whilst still awake. A focused mind, a future to claim—now I am back to myself once again.

RUNAWAY LIFE

My life ran away before my eyes. The things I know … the things I have seen. I closed it down and then opened it up. I do not want the memory, do not want the pain. The stress ignited my creativity like a firecracker. It rained black, but all it did was wash away the doubts. Remember the pain to feel the rain.

Far away from home. I took the risk to stand on the edge— to save my soul and even the odds.

I believe in the good deep within. It is the time to shine—to bring out the shooting star within. I know the truth that hides behind my eyes.

I know it is time to control and have the life I really want.

ALIVE

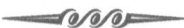

I feel so high. I come alive after the drudgery of the black abyss. I really need to be gently caught, but I enjoy the rush. The feeling is so good after being so forlorn and low.

Up and down. I am enjoying the bounce of going up. It starts off fun—a welcome feeling I cannot resist. Everything is beautiful—a warm, cosy feeling. I seem to chatter too much.

Energised and high, I feel I could touch the sky. The perfect day in a dreamy haze. A surreal dream, but I am still awake. I love the night; the stars are alive as I stand under a moonlit sky. I just feel so good.

I am sleeping less; the morning calls of the birds wake me up. But I must beware; if I become too elated, I will end up crushed, irritable, restless. My anxiety is up, and I am filled with paranoia as I take in too much.

It is often a fleeting feeling where I gently bounce. If it gets too much, time to ring the doctor for meds to bring me down.

Back to reality, but I loved the ride. But as a fleeting feeling it feels so nice.

BLACK SHADOWS

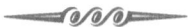

Screaming, breathing, dying, crying.

Hanging on to breath, too tired to wake, too scared to sleep.
Black shadows fleeting. Too tired, too trapped to move. Not
dying tonight. Pulling back to the light I need to survive.

Praying, screaming, crying, dying.

What deceit, what shame. Fleeing the pit of vipers. Trying
to find the cradle of light to save my life—the elixir of life,
pure and undefiled.

Cup of life, save my life. Save my soul, eyes wide open but
mind closed shut. The cross is my saviour: the bringer of
life—the destroyer of darkness, pulling me back to the light.
A prayer to end became the prayer of life.

MENTAL ILLNESS

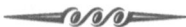

Mental illness is Iike childhood fantasy that becomes blurred with reality. Inanimate becomes animate. It is a scary world where dreams become reality—a nightmare that knows no bounds. It is a narrative on life where symbolism becomes reality and reality has no limits. I now know my reality, but the dreams were inspiring.

A BOND

My life caved in. I was lost in a sea of disbelief. Everything I knew was different. There was a mind malfunction, a malicious dream, a terrible fantasy that was not real. But everything seemed so true. I believed the nightmare—a twisted dream that felt so true.

Paranoid delusions broke my trust. I became lost in this contorted view. The world was against me. Family became foes; friends became plotters. The actions of others were interwoven into my nightmarish dreams—a scary place where I was on my own.

Mental anguish, fear, and loathing. How did I become so distorted? The plot thickened. I was frightened for my life, with a paranoid view that skewed my mind. I needed help, but everything felt so true. Unsafe and dazed, my friends and family were mystified. The doctors came. Time to mend my broken mind.

A spell in hospital and a new drug, but I still felt the same. My mum, a saint, fought in my corner, and the paliperidone was increased. She was always by my side, even though I lost my trust in all. She was my companion no matter how much I rejected or accused. The increase worked; the delusions ceased and lost their hold. I was lifted from the darkness of my mind's abyss.

My mum, a truly wonderful human being, never faltered or rejected me as my madness spun its web of deceit. The monsters were a figment of my mind. Paliperidone fixed my anguish and delivered me to a better place.

Three years on and I am still well. I now have a life, the land of the ethereal kingdom with visions and dreams a distant memory. The paranoid delusions that took such a hold no longer confuse what is real.

A lasting feeling is my love of my mum throughout this test—an unbreakable bond. I am now a stronger person who feels true joy, but this is a special thank you to Mum.

THE DAGGER AND THE SERPENT

I am the dagger the serpent entwines. I am the heart that owns the soul. Claim my soul; take my light as our shadows embrace. Entwine my purple heart. I am the staff whose rifts were healed by the strong hand that has clasped my soul.

He is the soul shaker; the devil may cry. My heart has been won by the silent one—the key to the throne, the key to my besotted heart. He is the soul shaker, the heart taker, the barbed wire ripped away from my crushing heart. The rose so young has become the rose betrothed to the magical, mythical one.

Red for danger, red for passion. Pink for the truest of loves cast amongst the shadows as we embraced under the stars so bright. Longevity of love. The dark is my smile, the emerald in my eye, the breath to my voice, the light in my heart—the love that perfected my life.

My life, once a crown of thorns, now has a golden hue, beset with the deepest sunset on the longest night. A solstice of love, an ethereal dream surreal and sun-kissed but dark like the mist, cold and eerie but as joyous as the first call of spring.

The reaper of love, the reaper of my heart. An immortal love. An eternity together as in the tombs of old. A story of love. A noble heart that has reaped my once solitary soul. The dagger and the serpent, which are entwined together forever in a clasp-like hold.

WHEN I LOST MY MIND

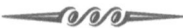

There was a time I lost my mind. My heart was full of disbelief. My partner died; I did not feel. It was just a descent into a land of misbelief. Paranoia, voices, monsters beckoning at my door, distorted visions … I lost my grip on reality. Dazed and confused, I turned in on myself, the focus my skewed thoughts.

The paranoia destroyed my trust. Lonely and scared, I rejected my family, who I thought were up to their worst. My mum, my saviour, never left my side, though she did not understand. It felt so real; the delusions took hold. She called the doctors, and to hospital I went. I was eventually discharged, with paliperidone as my new drug regime. But I was still plagued by thoughts inside and outside my mind. Mum took up the cause and told the professionals I was still not cured. The paliperidone was upped to the maximum dose.

The haze cleared from my mind. I no longer felt confused; a fog was lifted from my mind. My illness went, but I wanted to hide. My behaviour had been so odd; embarrassed, I did not want to step out the front door. Taking small steps, I gradually began to confront the outside world. Three years have passed, and I am still well. I still have little ups and downs, but I have not lost insight or become seduced by a world of make-believe.

My inner reality reflects the real world, not a place of unreality with demons at my door. This was the story of a part of my life, but thanks to Mum and the mental health team, I am truly healed and enjoying life as it should be again.

AUTHOR'S NOTE

The author has dedicated this collection to her mum, who was her constant companion and supporter, whether she understood or not, during her breakdown. It is of interest to anyone who wants to further his or her understanding of mental illness. She hopes it will develop both understanding and compassion.